Total Knee REPLACEMENT

It's a Joint Effort

I0116436

Contents

This book is only to help you learn and should not be used to replace any of your doctor's advice or treatment.

Introduction

You and your doctor have decided that you will have knee replacement surgery. Many people, even famous athletes, have had this surgery and now lead active, normal lives. Total knee replacement will allow you to move more freely and with more comfort than you do now.

This booklet will help you know how your knee joint works and will teach you about surgery to replace it. You will also learn what to do before and after surgery to make sure you get the greatest benefit from your new knee.

On page 23, there is a list of questions you may wish to ask your doctor.

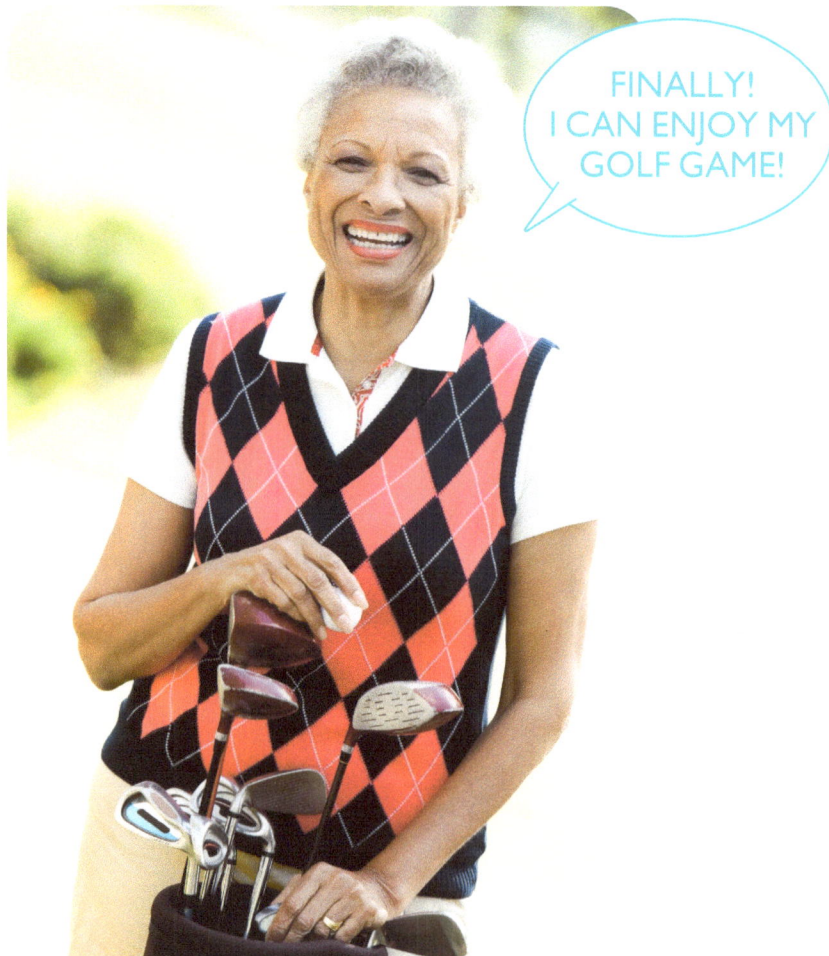

FINALLY! I CAN ENJOY MY GOLF GAME!

The thighbone's connected to the shinbone

The knee is the largest joint in the body. It is made of the thighbone (femur) and the shinbone (tibia). The knee cap (patella) sits in a groove on the femur and supports the tendons over the top of the knee.

Muscles, tendons and ligaments surround the knee joint. The ligaments and tendons keep the knee moving in the right direction.

A thin membrane (synovial membrane) surrounds the joint. It produces tiny amounts of fluid which lubricate ("oil") the joint. A shiny, smooth substance called *articular cartilage* covers the ends of the bones. The cartilage provides a smooth surface on your bones that makes movement easy and painless.

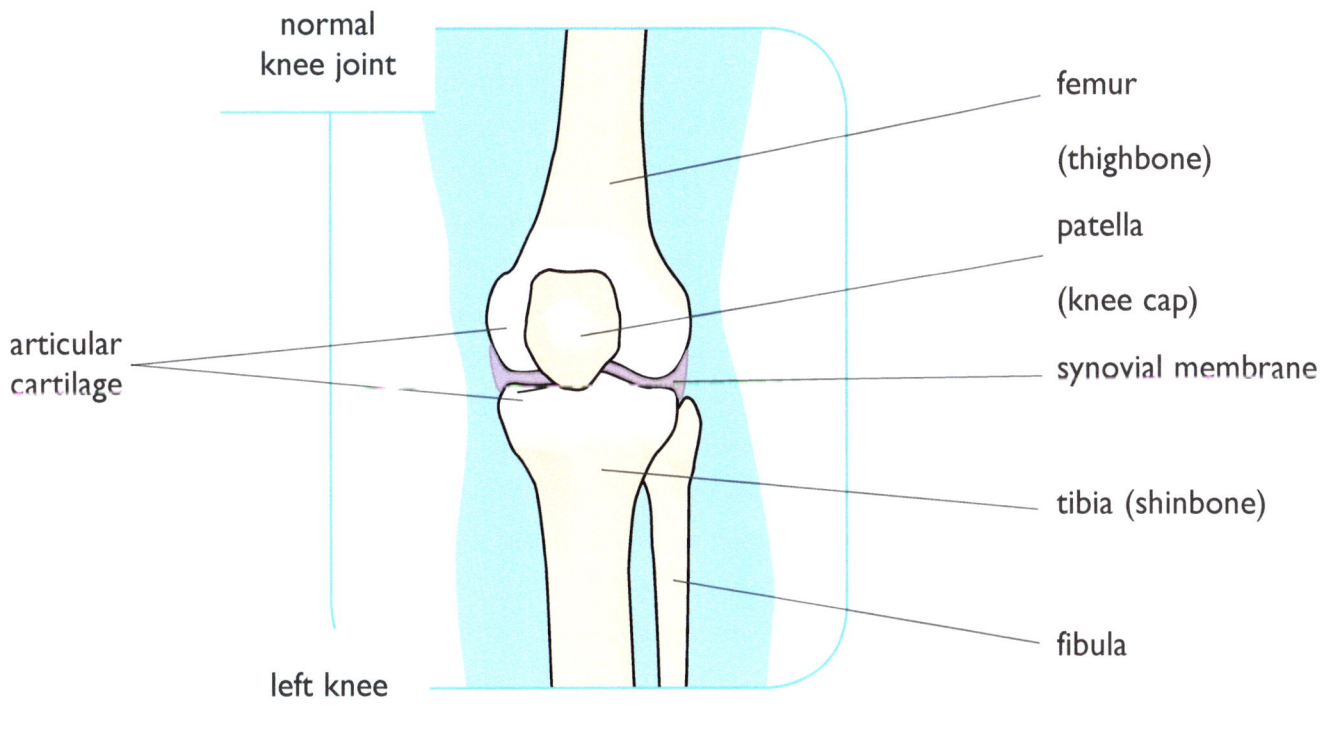

normal knee joint

femur

(thighbone)

patella

(knee cap)

synovial membrane

articular cartilage

tibia (shinbone)

fibula

left knee

hinge joint

The knee and elbow are types of **hinge joints.** These are joints made of two bones that meet end-to-end. The hinge action of the knee allows us to walk, run, climb steps, kneel and sit. Can you imagine how hard it would be to get into your car without bending your knees?

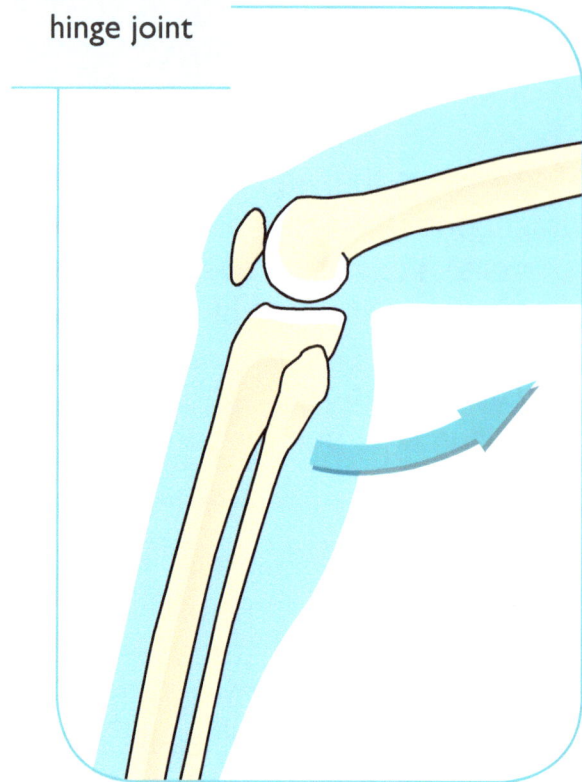

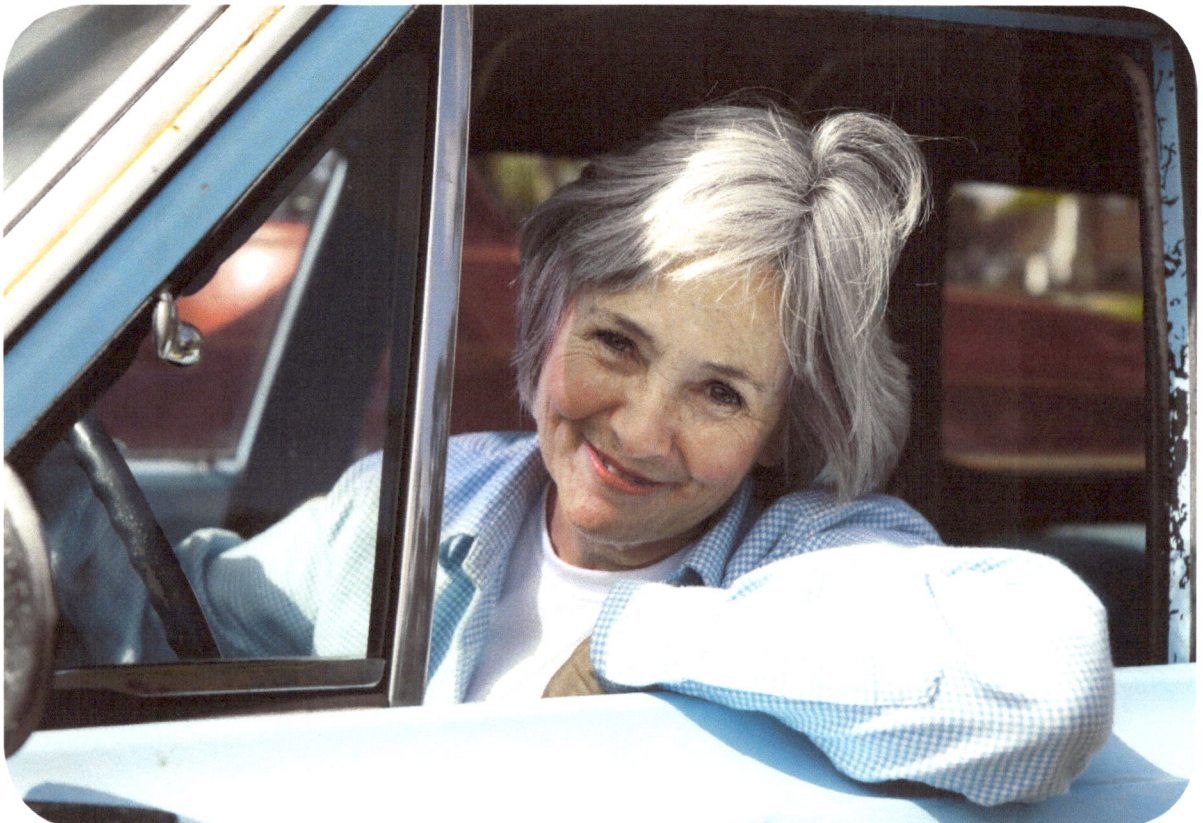

Some reasons for knee surgery

An injury, disease or normal aging can cause articular cartilage to become thin, rough or worn. When it does, the two bones begin to rub together. This results in a slow wearing away of the bone surface, which can cause pain and stiffness.

ARTHRITIS

Arthritis is a disease which affects over 43 million people. Arthritis is a "wearing away" of the joint surface.

There are 3 common types of arthritis that affect the knee:

- **Osteoarthritis** occurs as the articular cartilage thins due to age. This is not hereditary but does tend to run in families.

- **Rheumatoid arthritis** may affect many parts of the body including the synovial membrane in joints. The diseased membrane makes large amounts of fluid which thins the articular cartilage and makes the knee swell.

- **Traumatic arthritis** may occur at any age. This type of arthritis is caused from an injury to the joint which damages the articular cartilage.

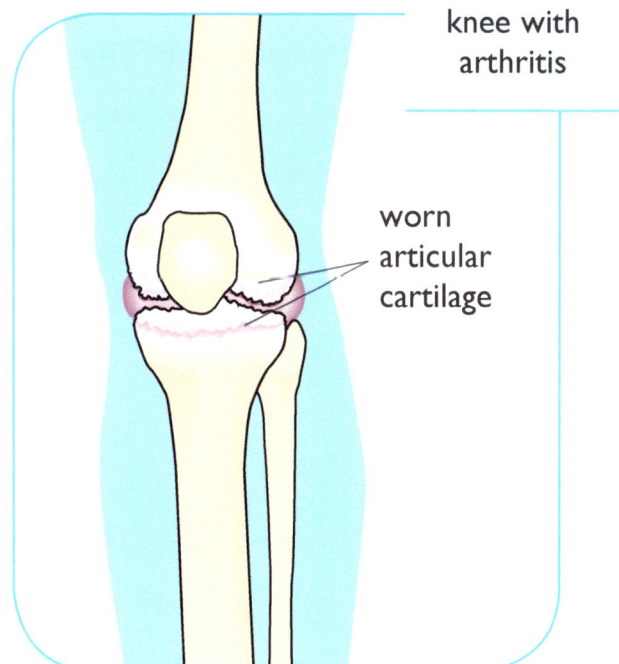

knee with arthritis

worn articular cartilage

Before your surgery

GETTING YOURSELF READY

Ask your doctor if the hospital offers pre-op classes. A class before surgery can do a lot to help you and your family get ready. Knowing what to expect can help ease your fears, as well.

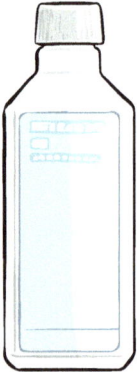

Arrange to have someone stay with you once you are discharged from the hospital.

You will most likely be asked to wash your entire body with a special soap for a number of days before your surgery. The soap is available over-the-counter in many brand names. This will help to prevent infection during your hospital stay.

If you smoke, now is the time to quit! Studies have shown that bones heal much faster in non-smokers.

Talk with your family doctor about your blood levels. You want to have a hgb (hemoglobin) level of over 12 gm/dL. If your level is too low, talk to your doctor about increasing your level by changing your diet.

Here are some other tips to get yourself ready:

- Prepare and freeze meals ahead of time so that you won't have to worry about cooking.

- Think about the room you are going to sleep in. Is it on the same floor as the bathroom and kitchen? If not, is the person caring for you able to carry meals up stairs?

- Put everything you might need on a bedside table so that it will be within easy reach. Make sure to include a phone and a lamp.

- Make sure you are eating a healthy diet and taking any supplements your doctor ordered.

GETTING YOUR HOUSE READY

There are a few small changes you can make in your home that can be a big help as you get over your surgery. So before you go to the hospital, it's a good idea to check around the house to see if changes are needed to make your recovery more comfortable.
To check around your house, sit:

- on the side of your bed

- in your favorite chair

- on the sofa

- on the toilet

- in the seat of your car

Is it hard to stand up after sitting down? If it is, you may want to change the height of your seat. You can raise the seat of a chair with pillows. You will find it much easier to get up from a sitting position or to sit down, if the seat is high. You can also use a chair with arms, so you can push up.

For more things that may help, see pages 19 and 20.

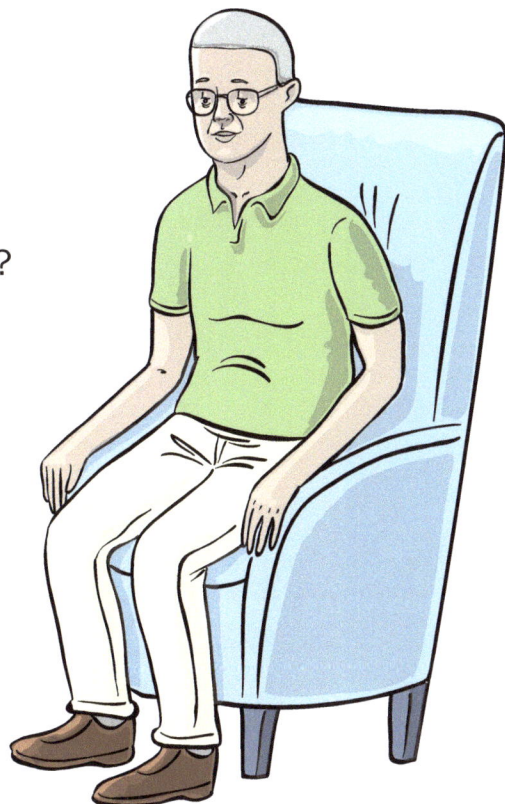

GETTING READY FOR THE HOSPITAL

When you go to the hospital take these with you:

☐ a list of all medicines you take
(including over-the-counter)

☐ a list of any allergies you have (to food, clothing,
medicine, etc.) and how you react to each one

☐ glasses, hearing aids and any other items you
use each day

☐ grooming items such as shampoo, toothpaste,
deodorant, etc.

☐ loose fitting shoes and shirt to wear for therapy

☐ knee length robe or cover-up for walking
in the halls

☐ shoes with closed in heels and non-slip soles

☐ walker or crutches (if you already
have them at home)

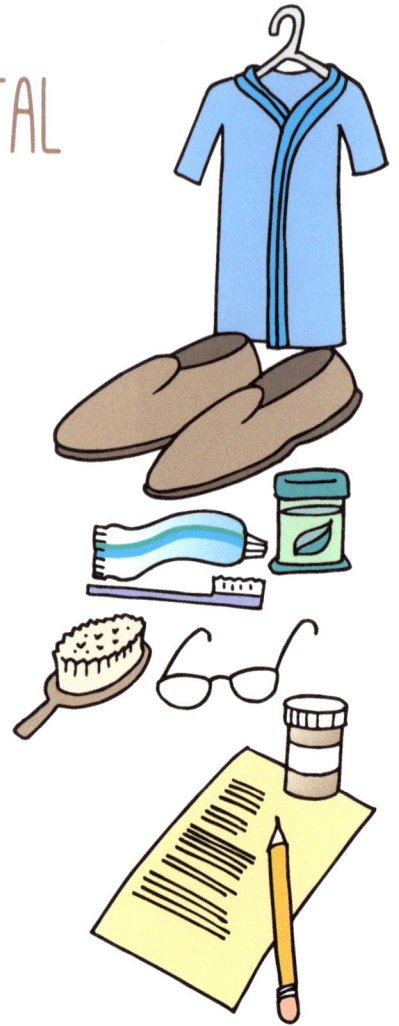

⭐ Many pain medicines can cause
constipation. Prepare now - learn
about changes you can make to
your diet in case this happens.

⭐ Put your name on everything
you take to the hospital.

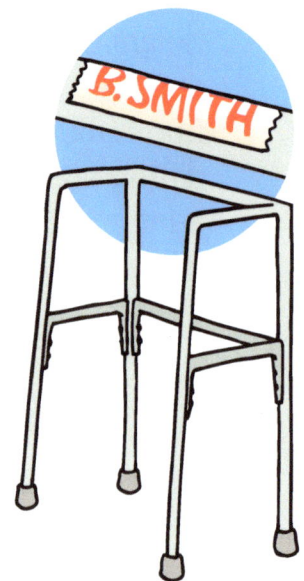

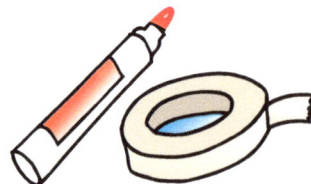

CONSENT FORM

Before surgery you must sign a consent form. This is a legal paper that says your doctor has told you about your surgery and any risks you are taking. By signing this form, you are saying that you agree to have the operation and know the risks involved. Ask your doctor any questions you may have about the operation and the results before signing this form.

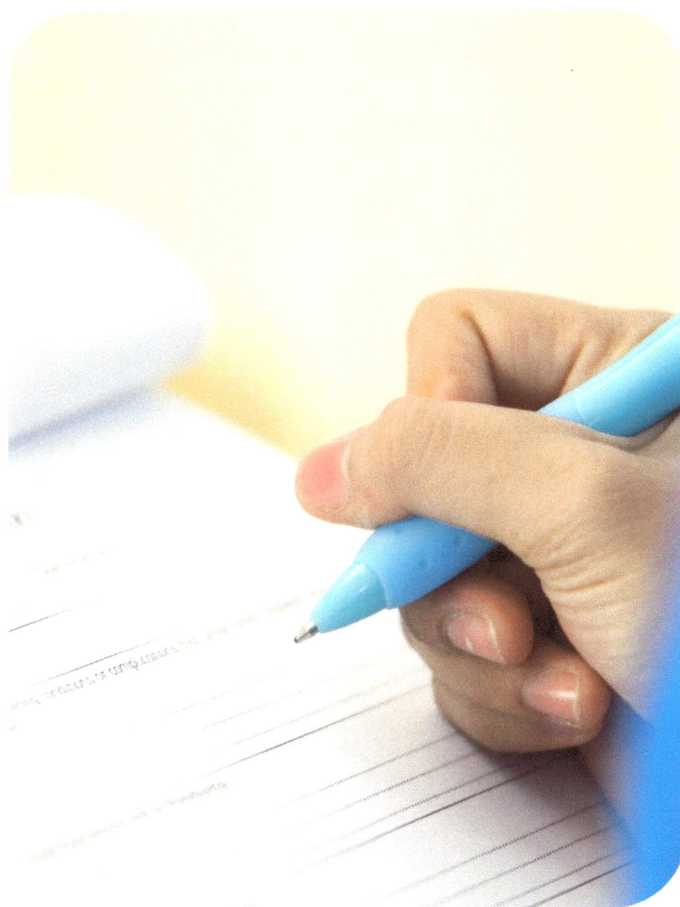

TESTS BEFORE SURGERY

Most people will have an ECG (heart tracing), a chest X ray and blood tests before surgery. Your orthopaedic surgeon may have you see your family doctor for a checkup. It is important that your blood levels be within a certain range before surgery. Your surgeon will review the results of these tests to make sure you are healthy and ready for surgery.

THE NIGHT BEFORE SURGERY

Many surgeons prefer that you don't eat or drink after midnight. Check with your doctor or nurse about this. If you take insulin, heart or blood pressure pills on a daily basis, discuss this with your doctor or nurse. They will make sure you do not miss any medicines that you need.

The morning of surgery

You will be asked to remove:

- dentures, hearing aids

- hairpins, wigs, etc.

- jewelry

- glasses, contact lenses

- nail polish

- all underwear

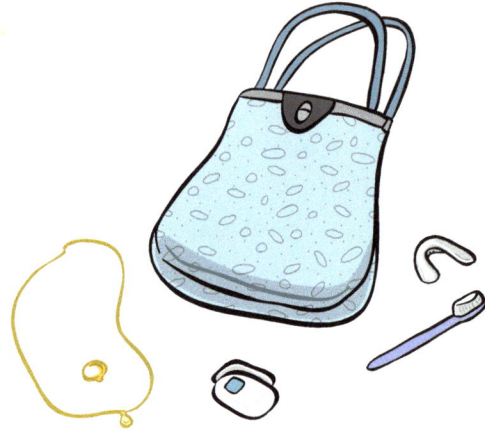

Have your family keep your things for you during surgery.

You will be able to visit with your family before leaving your room. You will be dressed in a hospital gown (nothing else). You should use the bathroom before you are taken to the operating room. You will ride on a stretcher (a bed with wheels) to the operating room. Once you are in the operating room, your knee will be scrubbed well with a special soap.

After you go to surgery, someone will show your family where to wait. From time to time, a member of the surgical team will update your family on your progress. Most of the time, knee surgery lasts from 45 minutes to 3 hours. You will also spend some time in the recovery room after surgery, so your time in the surgical area can be as long as 3 to 6 hours. Your doctor will tell you about how long your surgery will take. When the surgery is complete, the doctor will go to the waiting area and give your family a report.

While you are in surgery

Many people are in the operating room with you. Each hospital has its own routine, but these are some of the people who may be there:

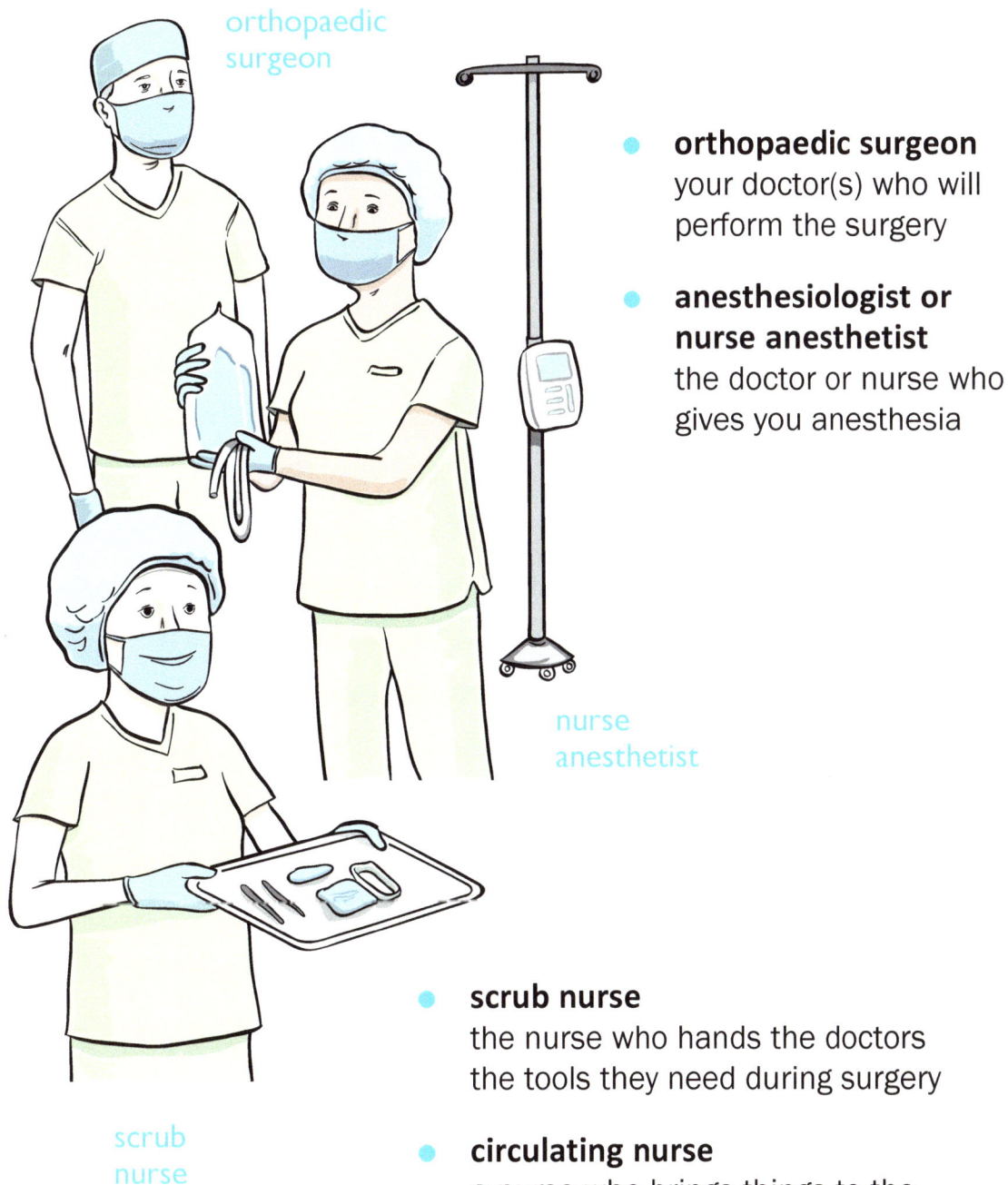

orthopaedic surgeon

nurse anesthetist

scrub nurse

- **orthopaedic surgeon**
  your doctor(s) who will perform the surgery

- **anesthesiologist or nurse anesthetist**
  the doctor or nurse who gives you anesthesia

- **scrub nurse**
  the nurse who hands the doctors the tools they need during surgery

- **circulating nurse**
  a nurse who brings things to the surgical team

Your surgeon and the anesthesiologist or nurse anesthetist will help you choose the best anesthesia to have. No matter what type of anesthesia you have, rest assured that you will not feel pain during the surgery. The types of anesthesia* you may have are:

- **general**
  You are put to sleep.

- **peripheral nerve block**
  Medicine will be injected around the nerves to make part of your body numb. This can be used on surgery for the upper or lower body.

- **epidural**
  You are numbed from the waist down with medicine injected into your back. (This is also used for women giving birth.)

- **spinal**
  Much like epidural, you are numbed from the waist down from medicine injected into your back.

An **intravenous tube (IV)** is placed in your arm. This lets your doctor replace fluids lost during surgery and give you pain medicine, antibiotics and any other medicines you may need.

A **catheter** (tube) may be placed in your **bladder.** This lets your health team keep up with your fluid intake and output. The catheter is most often removed the day after surgery.

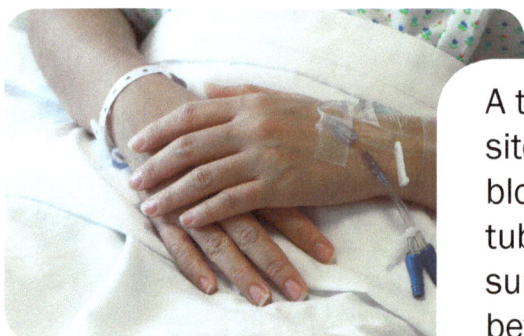

A third tube may come from your bandage site. This is a drain tube that helps reduce blood and fluid buildup at the incision. This tube will be removed 2 to 3 days after surgery. All of your tubes will be removed before you leave the hospital.

*Anesthesia may cause nausea. Extreme cases of nausea can be treated with medicine.

Your new knee

patellar replacement

tibial replacement

femoral replacement

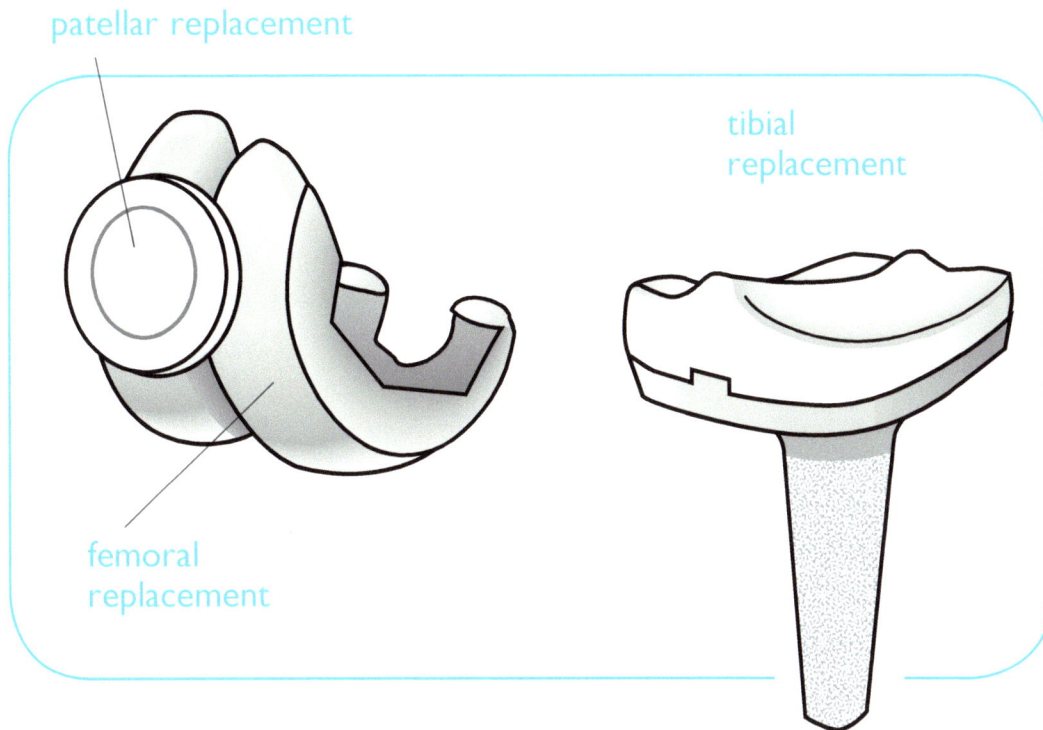

The surfaces of your knee joint will be removed, and a new metal and plastic prosthesis will be inserted.

The **femoral replacement** is metal and covers the end of the thighbone. The **tibial replacement** has a metal stem with a plastic tray which glides on the metal femoral piece. The **patellar replacement** is plastic and glides in the groove of the femur. The incision is closed with stitches or staples, a bandage is put on, and you are taken to a recovery room.

After surgery

THE RECOVERY ROOM

After surgery* you will spend a period of time in recovery. (The length of time can vary from person to person. It's usually between 1 and 3 hours.) Here, your blood pressure and heart rate are watched very closely. You will have a mask over your face to get oxygen. Later, you will be taken to your hospital room.

RETURNING TO YOUR HOSPITAL ROOM

Pain

Talk with your doctor **before** surgery about your pain medicine options. There are many new medicines and techniques to help you be more comfortable after surgery. You may receive pain medicine through your IV, through the epidural, in shots or pills or directly into the knee.

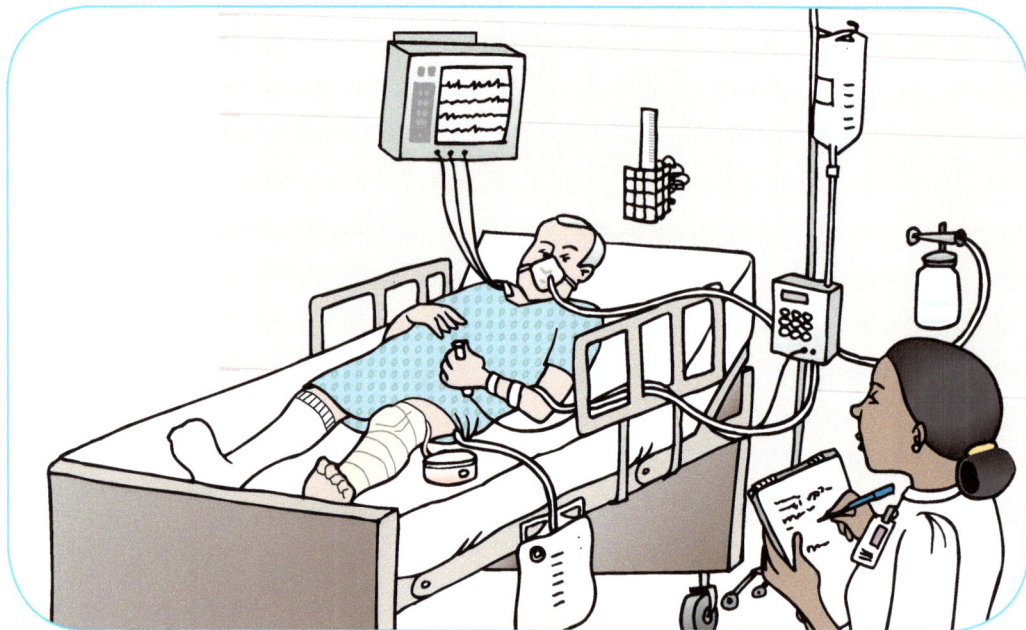

*You may not remember much about the surgery.

You will most likely experience some pain, but some people have very little. **It is very important that you begin moving around as soon as possible.** To do this you need to manage your pain. Do not wait to tell someone if you are hurting. Waiting may make it harder to relieve the pain. With proper management you can do **exercises and walk.** This is **important to your recovery.**

Your nurse or doctor may use a pain scale to measure the amount of pain you are in. This helps to figure out how well medicines and/or treatments are working. The scale may come in the form of a list of numbers, with or without pictures.

Usually, your pain is rated on a scale between 0 and 10, where 0 is no pain and 10 is the strongest pain. Your pain treatment is adjusted according to the level of pain you are in. So, be honest.

Pain scale

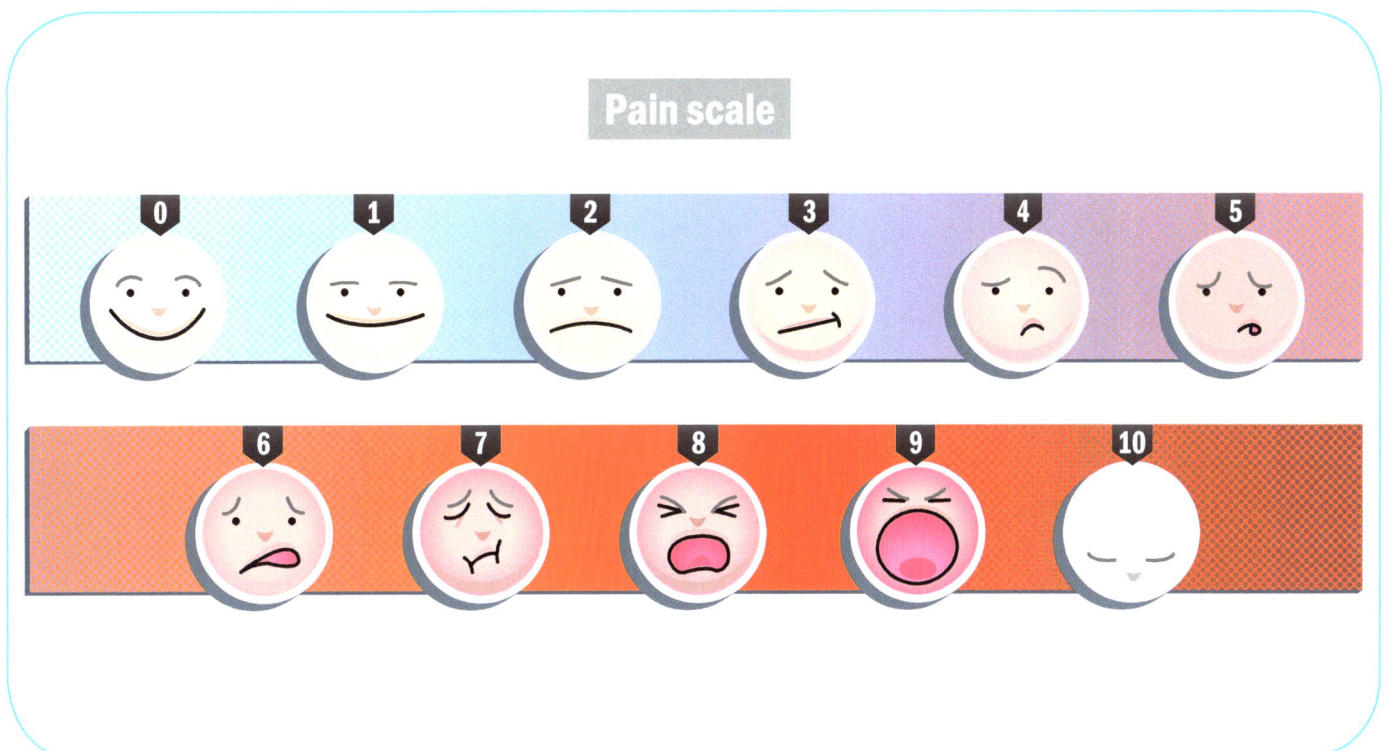

BREATHING

Right after your surgery, it will seem as if your nurse is always reminding you to take deep breaths and cough. **It is very important that you do this at least every 2 hours.** Deep breathing can help prevent pneumonia or other problems that can slow down your recovery and lengthen your hospital stay.

Your doctor may want you to use a device called an incentive spirometer. This device helps you breathe in and out the right way. Using it regularly and correctly can help keep your lungs clear.

Keep cylinder "floating" as you breathe in

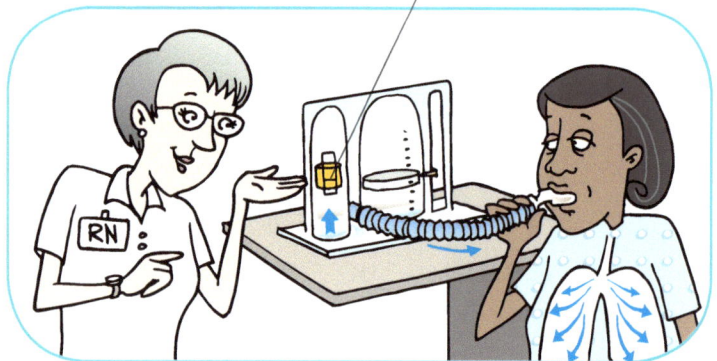

MOVEMENT

Most people begin exercising their knee the day of, or the day after surgery. A PT will work with you on specific exercises to make your leg and new knee stronger.

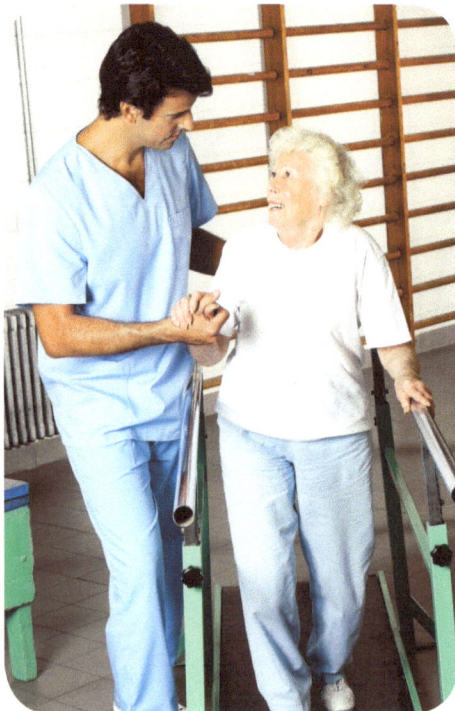

MOVEMENT (CONTINUED)

As you begin to move about in your room, you will notice your toilet seat and chair are raised. This is to make it easier for you to get up and down from a sitting position.

Moving around helps prevent blood clots after surgery. While you are in the hospital, the health care team will encourage you to get out of bed and walk often. When you go home, it is still very important that you walk often because you are still at risk for blood clots for several weeks after surgery.

BEFORE YOU LEAVE THE HOSPITAL

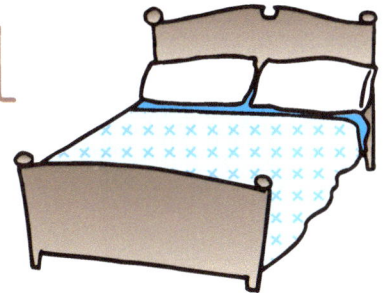

You will learn how to:

- get in and out of bed by yourself

- walk down the hall using your walker or crutches

- get in and out of the shower by yourself

- manage steps at home

- get in and out of your car

- do your exercise program by yourself

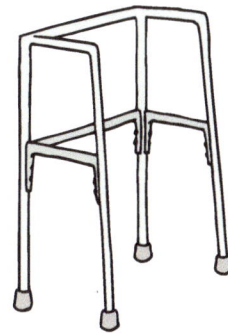

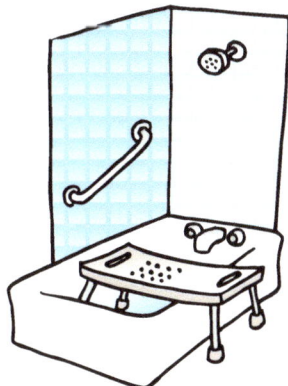

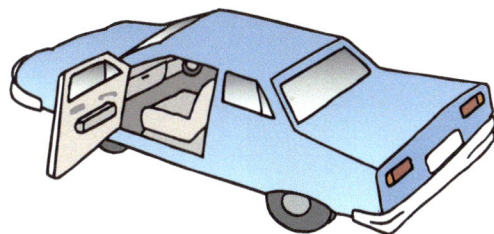

Preventing blood clots

Blood clots are the most common complication after total knee surgery. DVT (deep vein thrombosis) occurs when blood clots form in your abdomen, thigh or calf. If a clot breaks off and goes to your lungs, the blood supply to your lungs is cut off. This is called a pulmonary embolus and can be life-threatening.

The health team will remind you to do foot pumps every hour to push the blood out of your legs. Keep doing these after you go home. You are still at risk for getting blood clots weeks after joint replacement surgery. Walking is the best activity to prevent DVT.

You may have mechanical compression wraps on your legs or feet after surgery. These devices keep the blood from pooling in your legs. Your doctor may also order a blood thinning medicine to reduce the chance of blood clots.

Foot pumps

Pretend you are pushing down the gas pedal in a car.

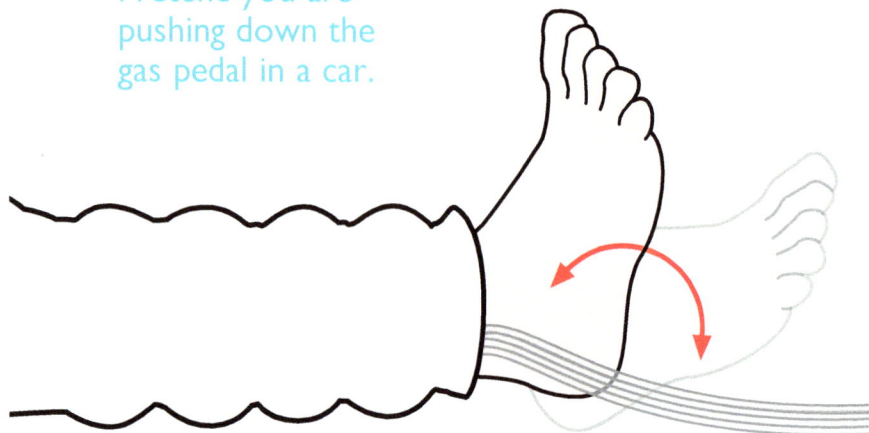

When you go home

Your doctor will decide how long you stay in the hospital. He may release you the day of surgery, or you could stay 1 to 2 days longer. It all depends on what your doctor decides is best for you. When you leave, all of the tubes will be out, and you may have a bandage on your knee. The swelling will most likely remain for a few weeks.

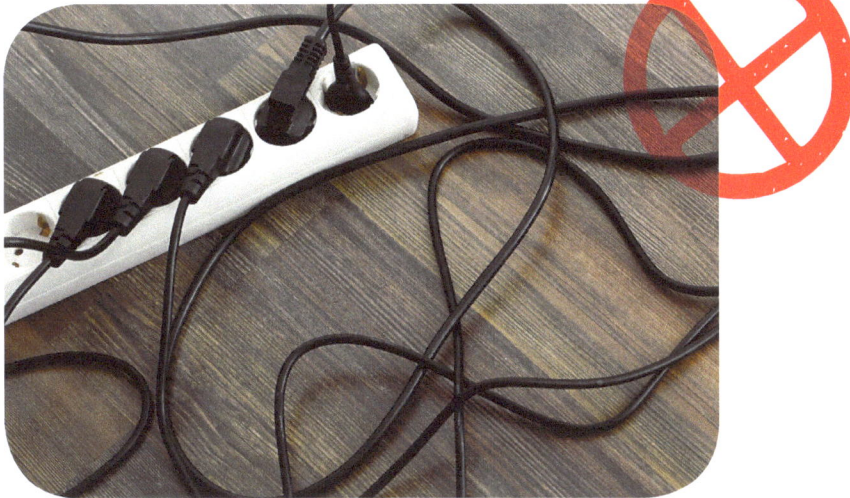

HOME SAFETY

Special care should be taken when you get home. Some common things in your home may now be a danger to you.

To prevent falls, remove or watch out for:

- long phone or electrical cords that lie across the floor

- loose rugs or carpet

- pets that run in your path

- water spills on bare floors

- wet bathroom tile or slippery floors

- ice or mildew on outdoor steps

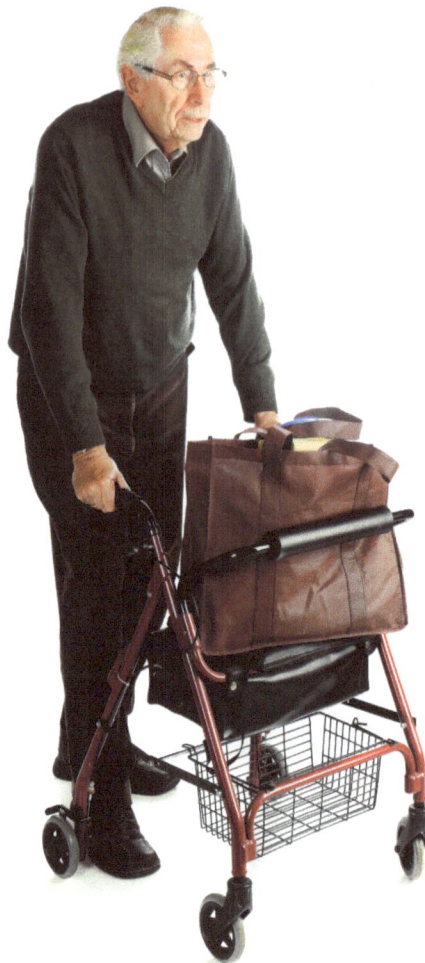

SPECIAL EQUIPMENT

You will not be able to move items, such as a cup of coffee, from one place to another while using a walker or crutches. A back pack, fanny pack or walker basket is a handy place to carry a thermos, sandwich or other item.

There is also other special equipment that can help you do things for yourself. **Dressing sticks** help you put on and take off your pants or underwear. **Long shoe horns** help you put on your shoes. **Elastic shoelaces** make your laced shoes into slip-on shoes. (A therapist can help you get these if you think they would be helpful.)

SPECIAL EQUIPMENT YOU MAY WANT TO USE AT HOME:

- ☐ Elastic shoelaces

- ☐ Back pack, fanny pack, walker basket

- ☐ Extra cushions, pillows

- ☐ Walker

- ☐ Crutches

- ☐ Cane

- ☐ Sock donner

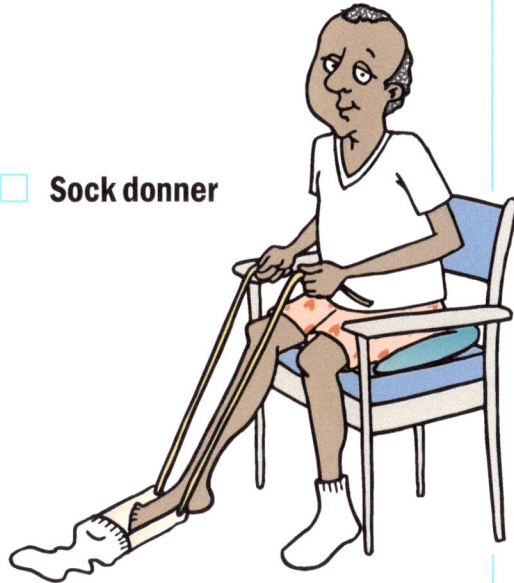

- ☐ Dressing stick

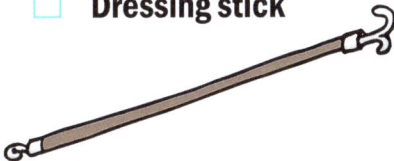

- ☐ Shoe horn

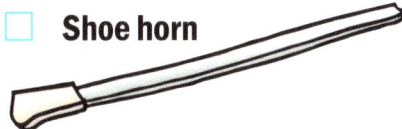

- ☐ Long-handled sponge

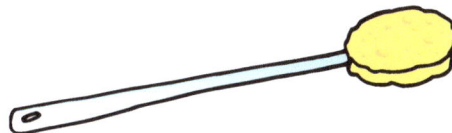

- ☐ Raised toilet seat

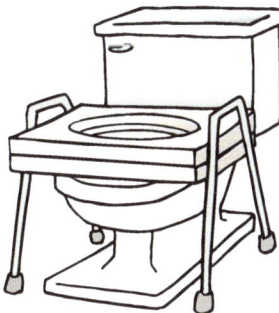

- ☐ Grabber

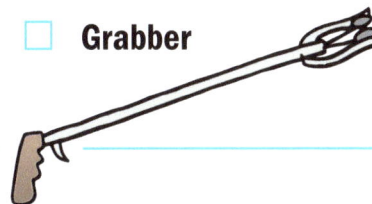

INCISION CARE

Your staples or stitches will be removed about 10 to 14 days after surgery. Your incision will heal, and the swelling and bruising will get better over the next 3 weeks. Look at your incision each day.

Call your doctor if you notice any of these:

- fever over 100°F/37.7°C
- drainage from incision
- redness around incision
- increased swelling around incision
- chest pain or congestion
- increased knee pain with activity or at rest
- problems with breathing
- calf pain or swelling in your legs

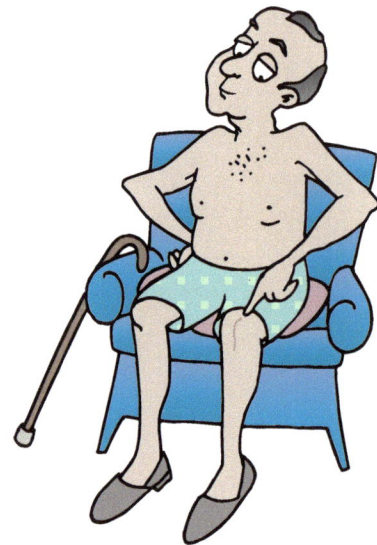

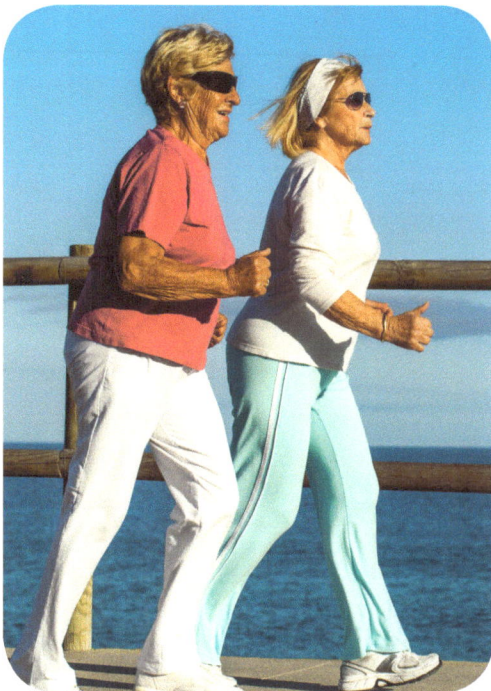

EXERCISE

When you get home, keep up the exercise program you learned in the hospital. Knee exercises should be done 2 to 3 times every day. Exercises are very important to help you get back the range of motion and strength in your knee. You will regain your strength and endurance as you begin to do your normal daily routine. Using ice for 20 minutes after every exercise session will reduce the swelling and pain in your knee.

LIVING WITH YOUR NEW KNEE

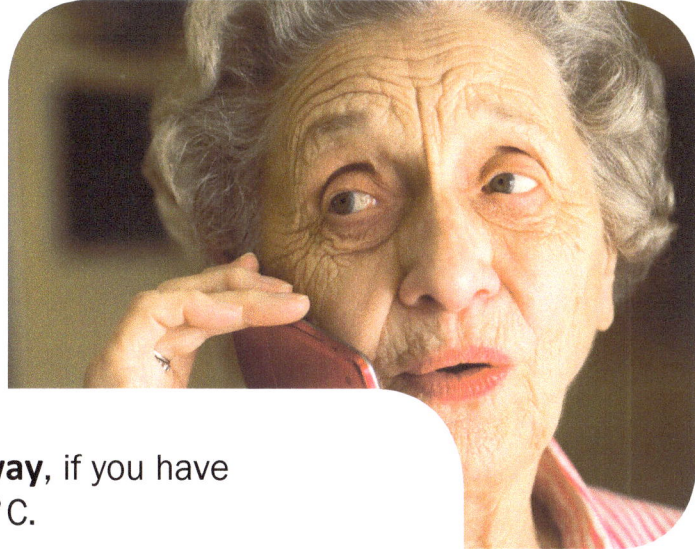

- **Call your doctor right away**, if you have a fever over 100°F/37.7°C.

- Keep your checkup appointments with your doctor. It is important to monitor the healing and function of your new knee.

- Your new knee is a large, foreign substance to your body. Germs from other areas can move to the new knee and cause infection. Call your family doctor at once if you have any signs of infection (urinary tract infection, abscessed teeth, etc.). Early treatment is needed.

- Tell your dentist and your doctor about your new knee BEFORE having your teeth worked on or having any procedure (such as cardiac cath, bladder exam, etc.) or surgery. Antibiotics may be needed before the procedure to prevent infection.

- Your new knee may set off metal detectors such as those in airports and some buildings. Your doctor can give you an ID card to carry in your wallet.

- Your new knee is designed to return you to low impact exercise such as walking, dancing, bike riding and golf. Talk with your doctor about the things you would like to do. High impact exercise such as jogging may cause your new knee to loosen.

Points to discuss with your doctor:

Take time now while your thoughts are fresh to write down any questions you wish to ask your doctor. Here are a few to help you get started.

What do you recommend I do to avoid constipation?

_____

Should I take my daily medicines on the day of surgery?

_____

What type of anesthesia is available? What do you recommend?

_____

How long will my family wait while I am in the operating and recovery rooms?

How will I get pain relief after surgery?

How long will I need to do my knee exercises and therapy?

_____

When can I drive?

When can I have sex?

Order this book from :

PRITCHETT & HULL ASSOCIATES, INC.
3440 OAKCLIFF RD NE STE 110
ATLANTA GA 30340-3006

or call toll free: 800-241-4925

This book is only to help you
learn, and should not be used
to replace any of your doctor's
advice or treatment.

Published and distributed by:
Pritchett & Hull Associates, Inc.

Printed in the U.S.A.

Your new knee

normal left knee

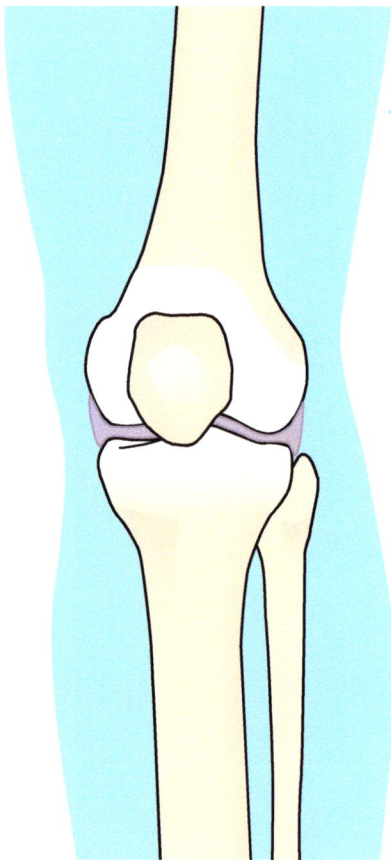

left knee replacement

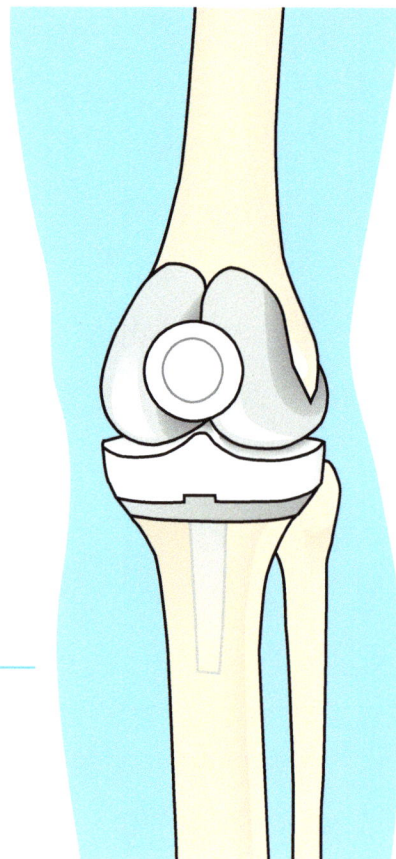

www.ingramcontent.com/pod-product-compliance
Lightning Source LLC
Chambersburg PA
CBHW060841270326
41933CB00002B/160